The Complete Boo

A Complete Collection of Thai Recipes to Boost Your Taste and Satisfy Your Appetite

Tim Singhapat

Table of contents

SOUTHEAST ASIAN ASPARAGUS

Ingredients:

- 1 cup toasted peanuts

- 1 pound asparagus, trimmed and slice into two-inch pieces

- 1 tablespoon sesame oil

- 1 teaspoon fish sauce

- 1 teaspoon toasted sesame seeds

Directions:

1. Heat the sesame oil in a big frying pan on moderate to high heat. Put in the asparagus and sauté for about three minutes.

2. Put in the fish sauce, sesame seeds, and peanuts. Sauté for two more minutes or until the asparagus is done to your preference.

Yield: Servings 4

ASIAN BURGERS

Ingredients:

- ¼ cup chopped basil

- ¼ cup chopped cilantro

- ¼ cup chopped mint

- 1 clove garlic, minced

- 1 pound ground beef or ground turkey

- 1 teaspoon sugar (not necessary)

- 2 tablespoons lime juice

- 3 shakes Tabasco

- 3 tablespoons bread crumbs

Directions:

1. In a moderate-sized-sized mixing container, mix all the rest of the ingredients.

2. Use your hands to gently mix the ingredients together and form 4 patties.

3. Season each patty with salt and pepper.

4. Grill the patties to your preference, approximately five minutes per side for medium.

Yield: Servings 4

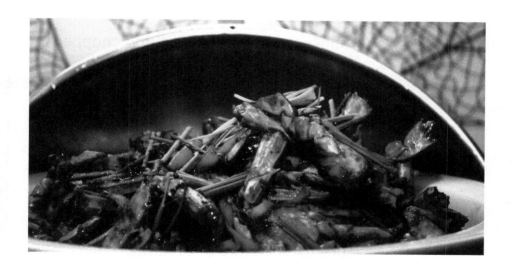

SHRIMP DIP

Ingredients:

- ½ serrano chili, seeded and minced

- ½ teaspoon grated lemon zest

- ½ teaspoon salt

- 1 tablespoon minced chives

- 5 tablespoons butter

- 8 ounces shrimp, cleaned and chopped

- Salt and freshly ground black pepper to taste

Directions:

1. In a moderate-sized-sized sauté pan, melt the butter on moderate heat. Mix in the chives, salt, chili pepper, and lemon zest; sauté for a couple of minutes.

2. Lower the heat to low and put in the shrimp; sauté for about three minutes or until opaque.

3. Move the mixture to a food processor and crudely purée. Sprinkle with salt and pepper.

4. Firmly pack the purée into a small container. Cover using plastic wrap, and place in your fridge for 4 hours or overnight.

5. To serve, remove the shrimp dip from the fridge and let it sit for five to ten minutes. Serve the dip with an assortment of crackers and toast points or some favorite veggies.

Yield: Approximately 1 cup

CHICKEN PIZZA

Ingredients:

- ¼— cup peanut or hot chili oil

  ½ cup crudely chopped dry-roasted peanuts 1
- cup chopped cilantro
- leaves

- 1 medium carrot, peeled and crudely grated

- 1 recipe Asian or Thai Marinade

- 1 unbaked pizza crust

- 1½ cups bean sprouts

- 1½ cups fontina cheese

- 1½ cups mozzarella cheese

Directions:

1. Put the chicken breasts in an ovenproof dish. Pour the marinade over the chicken, flipping to coat completely. Cover and place in your fridge for minimum 8 hours. Allow the

chicken to return to room temperature before proceeding.

2. Preheat your oven to 325 degrees. Bake the chicken for thirty to forty minutes or until thoroughly cooked. Take away the chicken from the oven and let cool completely. Shred the chicken into minuscule pieces; set aside.

3. Prepare the pizza dough in accordance with package directions.

4. Brush the dough with some of the oil. Top the oil with the cheeses, leaving a ½-inch rim. Evenly spread the chicken, green onions, carrot, bean sprouts, and peanuts on top of the cheese. Sprinkle a little oil over the top.

5. Bake in accordance with package directions for the crust. Remove from oven, drizzle with cilantro, before you serve.

Yield: 1 large pizza

THAI PASTA SALAD

Ingredients:

- ¼ teaspoon ground ginger

- ½ teaspoon red pepper flakes

- 1 clove garlic, minced

- 1 cup bean sprouts

- 1 cup rice wine vinegar

- 1 tablespoon brown sugar

- 1 tablespoon soy sauce

- 1½ cups thinly cut Napa cabbage or bok choy 1½ cups thinly cut red
- cabbage 2 medium
- carrots, shredded

- 2 tablespoons vegetable oil

- 2 tablespoons water

- 3 green onions, trimmed and thinly cut

- 3 tablespoons smooth peanut butter

- 8 ounces dried bow tie or other bite-sized pasta

Directions:

1. Cook the pasta in accordance with package directions. Drain and wash under cold water. Put the pasta in a big mixing container and put in the green onions, carrots, and cabbage.

2. In a small mixing container, meticulously mix all the rest of the ingredients except the sprouts.

3. Pour the dressing over the pasta and vegetables; cover and place in your fridge for minimum 2 hours or overnight.

4. Just before you serve, throw in the bean sprouts.

Yield: Servings 8–12

THAI-FLAVORED GREEN BEANS

Ingredients:

- ½ cup chopped cilantro

- 1 rounded tablespoon shrimp paste

- 2 pounds French or regular green beans, trimmed and slice into bite-sized pieces

- 2 tablespoons vegetable oil

- 2 teaspoons minced garlic

- 3 tablespoons unsalted butter

Directions:

1. In a pot big enough to hold all of the beans, steam them until soft-crisp.

2. Drain the beans, saving for later cooking liquid. Cover the beans using foil to keep warm.

3. In a small container, whisk together the shrimp paste and vegetable oil.

4. In a big frying pan, melt the butter on moderate to high heat. Put in the garlic and sauté until golden. Mix in the shrimp paste

mixture and 1 tablespoon of the reserved cooking liquid.

5. Put in the reserved green beans, stirring to coat. Cook until thoroughly heated.

6. Take away the pan from the heat and toss in the cilantro.

Yield: Servings 6–8

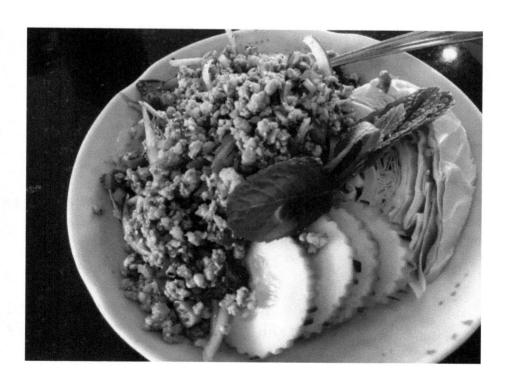

THAI-SPICED GUACAMOLE

Ingredients:

- 1 big plum tomato, seeded and chopped
- 1 small garlic clove, minced
- 1 tablespoon chopped onion
- 1 teaspoon chopped serrano or jalapeño chili
- 1 teaspoon grated gingerroot
- 1 teaspoon grated lime zest
- 1–2 tablespoons chopped cilantro
- 2 ripe avocados, pitted and chopped
- 4 teaspoons lime juice
- Salt and freshly ground black pepper to taste

Directions:

1. Put the avocado in a moderate-sized container. Put in the lemon juice and crudely mash.

2. Put in the rest of the ingredients and gently mix together.

3. Serve within 2 hours.

Yield: 2 cups

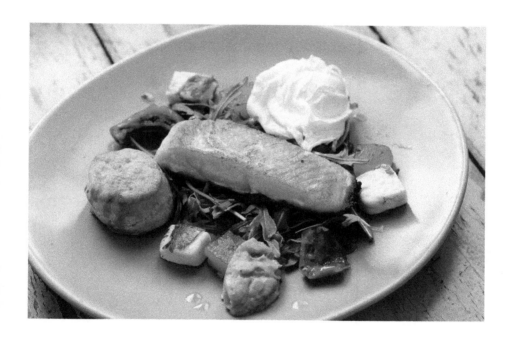

THAI-STYLE GRILLED PORK CHOPS

Ingredients:

- 1 cup fish sauce

- 2 (1-inch-thick) pork chops

- 2 tablespoons cream sherry

- 2 teaspoons brown sugar

- 2 teaspoons minced gingerroot

- 3 tablespoons rice vinegar

- garlic clove, minced

Directions:

1. In a small deep cooking pan, on moderate heat, bring the garlic, fish sauce, sherry, vinegar, brown sugar, and gingerroot to its boiling point. Turn off the heat and let cool to room temperature. (You can also put the marinade in your fridge to cool it.)

2. Put the pork chops in a plastic bag and pour in the marinade, ensuring to coat both sides of the chops. Allow the chops marinate at room temperature for fifteen minutes.

3. Pour the marinade into a small deep cooking pan and bring to a simmer on moderate to low heat. Cook for five minutes.

4. Grill the chops on a hot grill for five to six minutes per side for medium.

5. Serve the chops with the marinade sprinkled over the top.

Yield: Servings 2

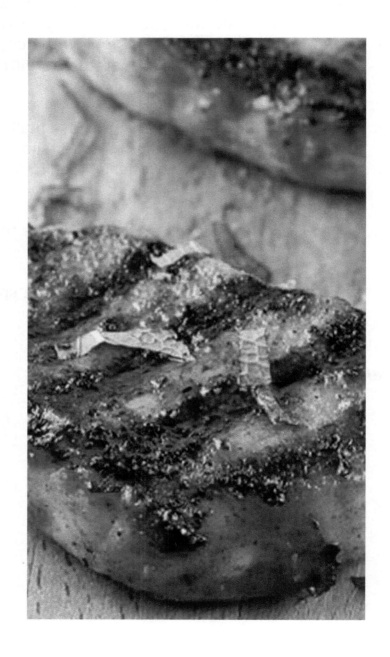

5 SPICED VEGETABLES

Ingredients:

- ¼ teaspoon crushed red pepper flakes

- ½ — ¾ teaspoon Chinese 5-spice powder

- ½ cup orange juice

- 1 cup carrot slices

- 1 pound mushrooms, cut

- 1 small onion, halved and thinly cut

- 1 tablespoon cornstarch

- 1 tablespoon vegetable oil

- 1–2 cloves garlic, minced

- 2 tablespoons soy sauce

- 2 teaspoons honey

- 3 cups broccoli florets

Directions:

1. In a small container, mix the orange juice, cornstarch, 5-spice powder, red pepper flakes, soy sauce, and honey; set aside.

2. Heat the vegetable oil in a wok or frying pan on moderate to high heat. Put in the mushrooms, carrots, onion, and garlic. Stir-fry for roughly 4 minutes.

3. Put in the broccoli and carry on cooking an extra 2 to 4 minutes.

4. Mix in the sauce. Cook until the vegetables are done to your preference and the sauce is thick, roughly two minutes.
5. Serve over rice noodles, pasta, or rice.

Yield: Servings 4

ALMOND "TEA"

Ingredients:

- ¼–½ cup sugar

- ½ teaspoon ground cardamom

- 2 cups milk

- 2 ounces pumpkin seeds

- 3 cups water

- 3 ounces blanched almonds

Directions:

1. Process the almonds, pumpkin seeds, cardamom, and half of the water in a blender or food processor until the solids are thoroughly ground.

2. Strain the almond water through cheesecloth (or a clean Handi Wipe) into a container. Using the back of a spoon, press

the solids to remove as much moisture as you can.

3. Return the almond mixture to the blender and put in the remaining water. Process until meticulously blended.

4. Strain this liquid into the container.

5. Mix the milk into the almond water. Put in sugar to taste.

6. Serve over crushed ice.

Yield: Servings 4–6

BANANA BROWN RICE PUDDING

Ingredients:

- ¼ cup water

- ½ teaspoon cinnamon

- ½ teaspoon nutmeg

- 1 (fifteen-ounce) can fruit cocktail, drained

- 1 cup skim milk

- 1 medium banana, cut

- 1 teaspoon vanilla extract

- 1½ cups cooked brown rice

- 2 tablespoons honey

Directions:

1. In a moderate-sized-sized deep cooking pan, mix the banana, fruit cocktail, water, honey, vanilla, cinnamon, and nutmeg. Bring to its boiling point on moderate to high heat. Lower the heat and simmer for about ten minutes or until the bananas are soft.

2. Mix in the milk and the rice. Return the mixture to its boiling point, decrease the heat again, and simmer for ten more minutes. Serve warm.

Yield: Servings 4–6

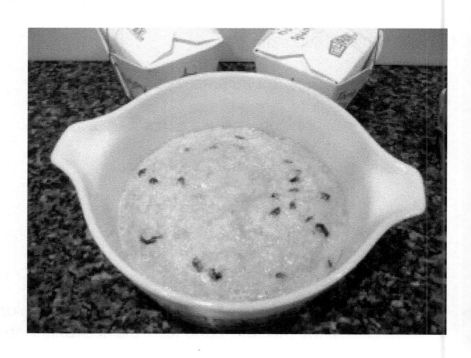

BASIC VIETNAMESE CHILI SAUCE

Ingredients:

- ½ teaspoon brown sugar

- 1 tablespoon lemon juice

- 1 tablespoon rice wine vinegar

- 2 cloves garlic, minced

- 2 dried red chilies, stemmed, seeded, and soaked in hot water until soft

- 2 tablespoons fish sauce

Directions:

1. Using a mortar and pestle, grind together the dried chilies and the garlic to make a rough paste.

2. Mix in the sugar until well blended. Mix in the rest of the ingredients.

Yield: Approximately ¼ cup

BEEF CAMBOGEE

Ingredients:

- ½ cup chopped peanuts

- 1 pound sirloin, trimmed, and slice into bite-sized pieces

- 2 cups bean sprouts

- 2–3 moderate-sized russet potatoes, peeled and slice into bite-sized pieces

- 5 cups Red Curry Cambogee (recipe on page 250)

Directions:

1. In a big deep cooking pan, bring the curry sauce to a simmer.

2. Put in the meat and potatoes and simmer until done to your preference, approximately twenty minutes to half an hour.

3. Decorate using the peanuts and bean sprouts.

Yield: Servings 4–6

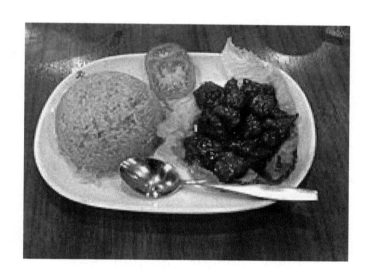

CAMBODIAN BEEF WITH LIME SAUCE

Ingredients:

- 1 tablespoon sugar

- 1 teaspoon water

- 1½ pounds sirloin, trimmed and slice into bite-sized cubes

- 2 tablespoons lime juice

- 2 tablespoons soy sauce

- 2 tablespoons vegetable oil

- 2 teaspoons freshly ground black pepper, divided 5–7
- cloves garlic, crushed

Directions:

1. In a container big enough to hold the beef, mix the sugar, 1 teaspoon of black pepper, soy sauce, and garlic. Put in the beef and toss to coat. Cover and let marinate for half an hour

2. In a small serving dish, mix the rest of the black pepper, the lime juice, and the water; set aside.

3. In a big sauté pan, heat the vegetable oil on moderate to high heat. Put in the beef cubes and sauté for about four minutes for medium-rare.

4. This dish may be served either as an appetizer or a main dish. For the appetizer, mound the beef on a plate lined with lettuce leaves with the lime sauce on the side. Use toothpicks or small forks to immerse the beef into the lime sauce. For a main dish, toss the beef with the lime sauce to taste. Serve with Jasmine rice.

Yield: Servings 4

CAMBODIAN-STYLE PAN-FRIED CHICKEN AND MUSHROOMS

Ingredients:

- ½ teaspoon grated ginger

- 1 cup water

- 1½ pounds chicken breasts and legs

- 2 tablespoons vegetable oil

- 2 teaspoons sugar

- 4 cloves garlic, crushed

- 6 ounces dried Chinese mushrooms

Directions:

1. Put the dried mushrooms in a container, cover with boiling water, and allow to soak for half an hour Drain the mushrooms and wash under cold water; drain again and squeeze dry. Remove any tough stems. Chop the mushrooms into bite-sized pieces; set aside.

2. Put the vegetable oil in a wok or big frying pan on moderate to high heat. Put in the

garlic and the ginger and stir-fry for a short period of time.

3. Put in the chicken and fry until the skin turns golden.

4. Mix in the water and the sugar. Put in the mushrooms.

5. Lower the heat to low, cover, and cook until the chicken is soft, approximately 30 minutes.

Yield: Servings 4–6

CARDAMOM COOKIES

Ingredients:

- ½ cup fine sugar

- 1 cup fine semolina

- 1½ teaspoons ground cardamom

- 3 tablespoons all-purpose flour

- 4 ounces ghee

Directions:

1. Preheat your oven to 300 degrees.

2. In a big mixing container, cream together the ghee and the sugar until light and fluffy.

3. Sift together the semolina, all-purpose flour, and cardamom.

4. Mix the dry ingredients into the ghee mixture; mix thoroughly.

5. Allow the dough stand in a cool place for half an hour

6. Form balls using roughly 1 tablespoon of dough for each. Put on an ungreased cookie sheet and flatten each ball slightly.

7. Bake for roughly thirty minutes or until pale brown.

8. Cool on a wire rack. Store in an airtight container.

Yield: 2 dozen cookies

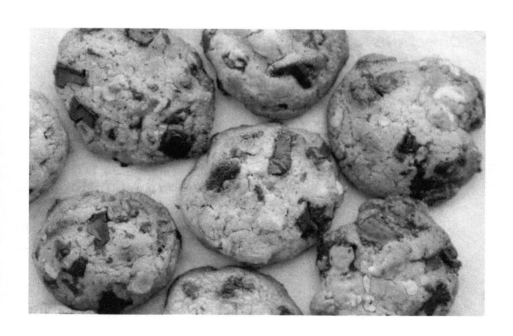

CHAPATI

Ingredients:

- 1 cup lukewarm water

- 1 tablespoon ghee or oil

- 1½ teaspoons salt

- 3 cups whole-wheat flour

Directions:

1. In a big mixing container, mix together 2½ cups of flour and the salt. Put in the ghee and, using your fingers, rub it into the flour and salt mixture.

2. Put in the lukewarm water and mix to make a dough. Knead the dough until it is smooth and elastic, approximately ten minutes. (Do not skimp on the kneading; it is what makes the bread soft.)

3. Form the dough into a ball and put it in a small, oiled container. Cover firmly using plastic wrap and allow it to rest at room temperature for minimum 1 hour.

4. Split the dough into golf ball–sized pieces. Using a flour-covered rolling pin, roll each ball out on a flour-covered surface to roughly 6 to 8 inches in diameter and -inch thick.

5. Heat a big frying pan or griddle on moderate heat. Put a piece of dough on the hot surface. Using a towel or the edge of a spoon, cautiously press down around the edges of the bread. (This will allow air pockets to make in the bread.) Cook for a minute.
Cautiously turn the chapati over and carry on cooking for 1 more minute. Chapatis must be mildly browned and flexible, not crunchy. Take away the bread to a basket and cover using a towel. Repeat until all of the rounds are cooked.

Yield: Servings 6–8

CHILIED COCONUT DIPPING SAUCE

Ingredients:

- ¼ cup fresh coconut juice

- 1 serrano chili, seeded and minced

- 1 tablespoon lime juice

- 1 teaspoon rice wine vinegar

- 1 teaspoon sugar

- 2 cloves garlic, minced

- 2 tablespoons fish sauce

Directions:

1. Bring the coconut juice, rice wine vinegar, and sugar to its boiling point in a small deep cooking pan. Turn off the heat and allow the mixture to cool completely.

2. Mix in the rest of the ingredients.

Yield: Approximately 1 cup

CUCUMBER RAITA

Ingredients:

- 1 teaspoon salt

- 1½ cups plain yogurt

- 1–2 green onions, trimmed and thinly cut

- 2 seedless cucumbers, peeled and slice into a small dice

- 2 tablespoons fresh mint

- Lemon juice to taste

Directions:

1. Put the diced cucumbers in a colander. Drizzle with salt and allow it to sit in the sink for fifteen minutes to drain. Wash the cucumber under cold water and drain once more.

2. Mix the cucumber, yogurt, green onions, mint, and lemon juice to taste.

3. Cover and place in your fridge for minimum 30 minutes. Check seasoning, putting in additional salt and/or lemon juice if required.

Yield: Approximately 4 cups

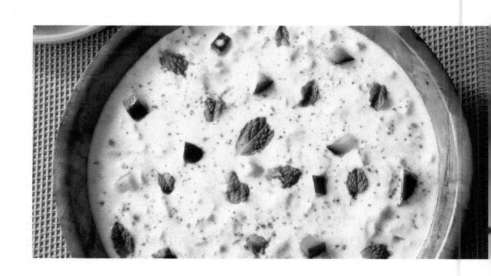

FRUIT IN SHERRIED SYRUP

Ingredients:

- 1 orange, peeled and segmented

- 1½ cups kiwi slices

- 2 cups fresh pineapple chunks

- 2 tablespoons dry sherry

- 2 tablespoons sugar

- 2 teaspoons lemon juice

- 4 tablespoons water

Directions:

1. In a small deep cooking pan using high heat, boil the sugar and the water until syrupy. Turn off the heat and let cool completely. Mix in the lemon juice and sherry; set aside.

2. In a serving container, mix the orange segments, the pineapple chunks, and the kiwi. Pour the syrup over the fruit and toss to blend. Place in your fridge for minimum 1 hour before you serve.

Yield: Servings 4–6

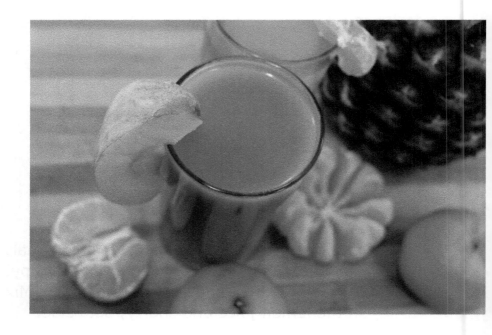

GARAM MASALA

Ingredients:

- 1 tablespoon whole black peppercorns

- 1 teaspoon whole cloves

- 2 small cinnamon sticks, broken into pieces

- 2 tablespoons cumin seeds

- 2 teaspoons cardamom seeds

- 4 tablespoons coriander seeds

Directions:

1. In a small heavy sauté pan, individually dry roast each spice on moderate to high heat until they start to release their aroma.
2. Allow the spices to cool completely and then put them in a spice grinder and process to make a quite fine powder.

3. Store in an airtight container.

Yield: Approximately 1 cup

HAPPY PANCAKES

Ingredients:

- ¼ cup mixed, chopped herbs (mint, cilantro, basil, etc.)

- ¼ teaspoon salt

- ½ cup bean sprouts

- ½ cup finely cut straw mushrooms,
- washed and patted dry 1 cup rice flour

- 1 tablespoon vegetable oil

- 1 teaspoon sugar

- 1½ cups water

- 2 eggs, lightly beaten

- 3 ounces cooked salad shrimp,
- washed and patted dry Chili
- dipping sauce

Directions:

1. In a moderate-sized-sized container, whisk together the rice flour, water, eggs, salt, and

sugar. Set aside and let the batter rest for about ten minutes.

2. Strain the batter through a mesh sieve to remove any lumps.

3. Put in the vegetable oil to a big sauté or omelet pan. Heat on high until super hot, but not smoking.

4. Pour the batter into the hot pan, swirling it so that it coats the bottom of the pan uniformly. Drizzle the mushrooms over the batter. Cover and allow to cook for a minute.

5. Drizzle the shrimp and bean sprouts uniformly over the pancake. Carry on cooking until the bottom is crunchy and browned.

6. To serve, chop the pancake into four equivalent portions. Drizzle with the chopped herbs. Pass a favorite dipping sauce separately.

Yield: Servings 4

HONEYED CHICKEN

Ingredients:

- ½ teaspoon Chinese 5-spice powder

- 1 (1-inch) piece ginger, peeled and minced

- 1 medium onion, peeled and slice into wedges

- 1 pound boneless, skinless chicken breasts, cut into bite-sized pieces

- 2 tablespoons fish sauce

- 2 tablespoons honey

- 2 tablespoons soy sauce

- 2 tablespoons vegetable oil

- 3–4 cloves garlic, thinly cut

Directions:

1. Mix the honey, fish sauce, soy sauce, and 5-spice powder in a small container; set aside.

2. Heat the oil in a wok on moderate to high. Put in the onion and cook until it just starts to brown.

3. Put in the chicken; stir-fry for three to four minutes.

4. Put in the garlic and ginger, and continue stir-frying for 30 more seconds.

5. Mix in the honey mixture and allow to cook for three to four minutes, until the chicken is glazed and done to your preference.

Yield: Servings 3–4

HOT NOODLES WITH TOFU

Ingredients:

- ½ pound Chinese wheat noodles

- ½ pound dried tofu, soaked in hot water for fifteen minutes and slice into 1-inch cubes

- ½ pound firm tofu, cut into 1-inch cubes ½ teaspoon yellow asafetida
- powder

- 1 bunch choy sum, chopped into 1-inch pieces

- 2 cups mung bean shoots or bean sprouts

- 3 tablespoons lemon juice

- 3 tablespoons minced ginger

- 3 tablespoons sambal oelek

- 3 tablespoons sesame oil

- 3 tablespoons soy sauce

- Vegetable oil for frying

Directions:

1. Cook the noodles firm to the bite in accordance with package directions. Wash under cold water and drain; set aside.

2. Heat approximately two inches of vegetable oil in a wok or big frying pan over moderate high heat. Put in the firm tofu cubes and deep-fry until golden. Using a slotted spoon, remove the tofu cubes to paper towels to drain; set aside.

3. Put in the dried tofu pieces and deep-fry them until they blister.
Remove and drain using paper towels; set aside.

4. In another wok or frying pan heat the sesame oil using high heat. Put in the ginger and stir-fry one minute.

5. Put in the asafetida and choy sum, and stir-fry until tender.

6. Mix in the soy sauce, sambal oelek, and lemon juice. Put in the noodles and tofu pieces. Stir-fry until hot, approximately 2 minutes more.

Yield: Servings 4

INDIAN-SCENTED CAULIFLOWER

Ingredients:

- ½ medium to big head of cauliflower, separated into florets and slice into pieces

- ½ teaspoon <u>Garam Masala</u>

- ½ teaspoon turmeric

- 1 (2-inch) piece ginger, peeled and minced

- 1 clove garlic, minced

- 1 teaspoon mustard seeds

- 1 teaspoon salt

- 3 tablespoons vegetable oil

- 3 tablespoons water

Directions:

1. In a deep cooking pan big enough to easily hold the cauliflower, heat the vegetable oil on moderate to high heat. Put in the mustard seeds and fry until they pop. Put in the garlic and the ginger; stirring continuously, cook until the garlic just starts to brown.

2. Mix in the turmeric. Put in the cauliflower pieces and toss to coat with the spice mixture.

3. Put in the water, cover, and allow to steam for 6 to ten minutes or until done to your preference.
4. Pour off any surplus water and drizzle with the garam masala.

Yield: Servings 2–4

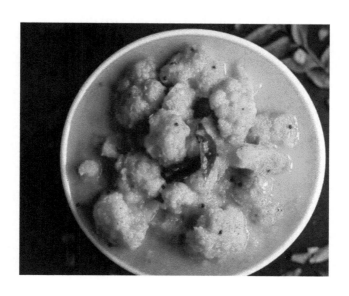

MANGO CHUTNEY

Ingredients:

- ½ ounce golden raisins

- ½ teaspoon black mustard seeds

- 1 cup water

- 1 tablespoon chopped ginger

- 1 tablespoon minced garlic

- 1 teaspoon cumin

- 1-2 red chili peppers, seeded and minced 2 big green
- mangoes, peeled and
- cut 2 cups sugar

- 2 cups white vinegar

- 2 teaspoons <u>Garam Masala</u>

- 3 teaspoons salt

- 4 ounces dried apricots or cherries

Directions:

1. Put all of the ingredients in a heavy-bottomed deep cooking pan. Heat to a simmer on moderate heat, stirring until the sugar dissolves.

2. Simmer for thirty minutes or until thick.

3. Seal in airtight jars.

Yield: Approximately 5–6 cups

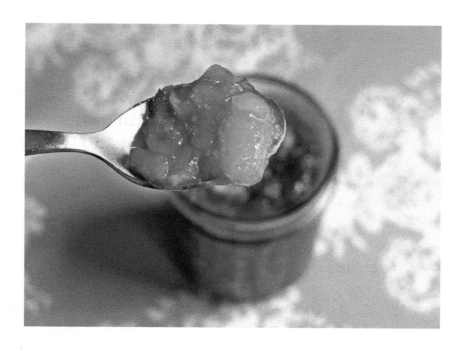

MINTED VEGETABLES

Ingredients:

- ½ cup vegetable broth

- 1 medium onion, cut into 1-inch pieces

- 1 red bell pepper, seeded and slice into 1-inch pieces

- 2 teaspoons vegetable oil, divided

- 3 cups broccoli pieces

- 3 cups thinly cut red cabbage

- 3–4 tablespoons chopped mint

- 4 medium carrots, peeled and slice into thin slices Salt and
- pepper to taste

Directions:

1. In a big frying pan, heat 1 teaspoon of vegetable oil on moderate to high heat. Put in the carrot slices, onion, and bell pepper; sauté for five minutes.

2. Put in the remaining teaspoon of oil, the broccoli, the cabbage, and the vegetable broth. Continue to sauté until the vegetables are done to your preference, approximately ten minutes for soft-crisp.

3. Sprinkle salt and pepper to taste. Mix in the chopped mint.

Yield: Servings 6

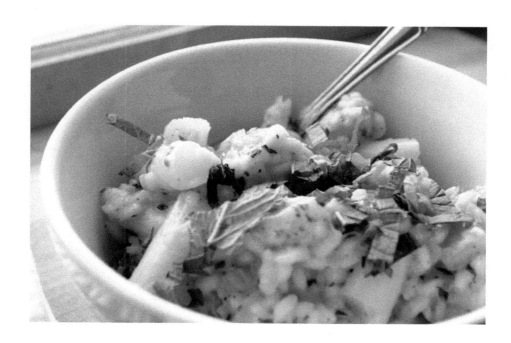

MULLIGATAWNY SOUP

Ingredients:

- 1 (1½-inch) cinnamon stick

- 1 (14-ounce) can coconut milk

- 1 jalapeño, seeded and cut

- 1 tablespoon ground cumin

- 1 tablespoon vegetable oil

- 2 medium onions, peeled

- 2 tablespoons ground coriander

- 2 teaspoons salt

- 2 teaspoons whole peppercorns

- 3 cloves garlic, peeled

- 3 pounds chicken wings

- 4 whole cloves

- 4–5 cups cooked rice

- 5 cardamom pods, bruised

- 6 cups chicken broth

- 8–12 fresh curry leaves

- Lemon juice to taste

Directions:

1. Put the chicken wings in a big soup pot. Cover the chicken with cold water.

2. Stick the cloves into 1 of the onions and put the onion in the pot with the chicken.

3. Put in the garlic, jalapeño, cinnamon stick, peppercorns, cardamom, coriander, cumin, and salt; bring the mixture to its boiling point, reduce to a simmer, and cook for two to three hours.

4. Allow the stock come to room temperature. Take away the chicken pieces from the broth and chop the meat from the bones. Set aside the meat.

5. Strain the broth.

6. Thinly slice the rest of the onion.

7. In a big sauté pan, heat the oil on moderate to high heat. Put in the onion slices and sauté until translucent. Put in the curry leaves and the broth. Heat to a simmer and allow to cook for five minutes.

8. Put in enough water to the coconut milk to make 3 cups of liquid. Put in this and the reserved meat to the broth. Heat the soup, but do not allow it to boil. Season to taste with additional salt and a squeeze of lemon juice.

9. To serve, place roughly ½ cup of cooked rice on the bottom of each container. Ladle the soup over the rice.

Yield: Servings 8–10

OYSTER MUSHROOM SOUP

Ingredients:

- ½ pound oyster mushrooms, cleaned and separated if large ½ stalk
- lemongrass, outer leaves removed, inner core finely chopped

- 1 tablespoon Tabasco

- 1 teaspoon sugar

- 2 tablespoons lemon juice

- 2–3 serrano chilies

- 3 (2-inch-long, ½-inch wide) pieces lime zest

- 4 cups vegetable broth

Directions:

1. In a big deep cooking pan, bring the vegetable broth and the Tabasco to its boiling point. In the meantime, crush the chilies with a mallet to break them slightly open: A good whack will do it.

2. Put in all of the rest of the ingredients to the boiling broth, reduce the heat, and simmer

until the mushrooms are cooked to your preference. Take away the chilies before you serve.

Yield: Servings 4

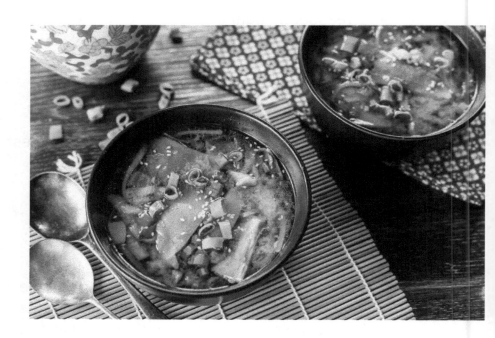

PENINSULA SWEET POTATOES

Ingredients:

- ¼ teaspoon salt

- 1 (14-ounce) can coconut milk

- 1 bay leaf

- 1 pound sweet potatoes or yams of varying varieties, peeled and slice into bite-sized pieces

- 1 teaspoon sugar

Directions:

1. Put the sweet potato pieces in a big deep cooking pan. Put in barely sufficient water to cover them, and bring to its boiling point. Put in the bay leaf and cook until the potatoes are tender. Take away the bay leaf and discard.

2. Mix in the sugar and salt. After the sugar has dissolved, remove the pan from the heat and mix in the coconut milk. Tweak the seasonings by putting in salt and/or sugar if required. Adjust the consistency by putting in more water and/or coconut milk.

Yield: Servings 4

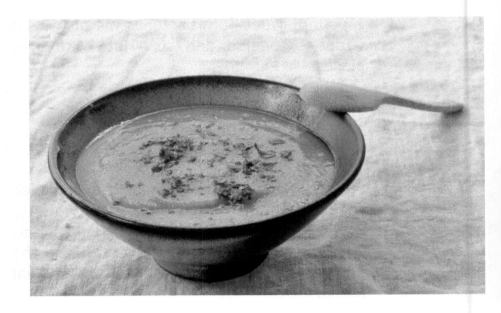

PORK MEDALLIONS IN A CLAY POT

Ingredients:

- ½ teaspoon ground black pepper

- 1 clove garlic, minced

- 1 cup water

- 1 tablespoon Black Bean Paste (Page 10)

- 1 tablespoon cornstarch

- 1 tablespoon Tamarind Concentrate (Page 20)

- 1 teaspoon rice wine

- 1 teaspoon sesame oil

- 2 pork tenderloins, trimmed and slice into ½-inch slices

- 2 tablespoons light soy sauce

- 2 tablespoons oyster sauce

- 2 tablespoons sweet (dark) soy sauce

63

- 2 tablespoons vegetable oil

Directions:

1. Prepare the marinade by combining the oyster sauce, light and dark soy sauces, Black Bean Paste, sesame oil, rice wine, black pepper, garlic, and cornstarch in a moderate-sized container.
2. Put in the pork slices to the container of marinade and toss to coat completely. Cover the pork and let marinate at room temperature for half an hour

3. Heat the vegetable oil in a wok on moderate to high heat. Put in the marinated pork and stir-fry for three to four minutes.

4. Move the pork to a clay pot or other ovenproof braising vessel.

5. Mix together the tamarind and water; pour over the pork.

6. Bake the pork in a 350-degree oven for about ninety minutes, until super soft.

Yield: Servings 4

POTATO SAMOSAS

Ingredients:

For the crust:

- ½ teaspoon salt

- 1½ cups all-purpose flour

- 4 tablespoons butter, at room temperature
- Ice water

- Vegetable oil for deep frying

For the filling:

- ¼ pound sweet peas, thawed if frozen

- ½ teaspoon chili powder

- ½ teaspoon turmeric

- 1 tablespoon ghee (see note) or oil

- 1 teaspoon salt

- 1¼ pounds russet potatoes, peeled

- 2 jalapeños, seeded and thinly cut

- 2 teaspoons mustard seeds

- 3 tablespoons chopped mint

- Lemon juice to taste

Directions:

1. To make the pastry crust: In a big container, sift together the flour and the salt. Using a pastry cutter, chop the butter into the flour mixture.

2. Put in the ice water, 1 tablespoon at a time, until a firm dough is achieved. You will probably use 5 to 6 tablespoons of water total. Knead the dough for roughly five minutes or until it is smooth and elastic. Put the dough in an oiled container, cover using plastic wrap, and set it aside while making the potato filling.

3. To make the filling: Bring a big pan of water to its boiling point. Put in the potatoes and cook until fairly soft. Drain the potatoes and let them cool until they are easy to handle. Cut them into a small dice; set aside.

4. In a big frying pan, heat the ghee on moderate to high heat. Put in the mustard seeds and sauté until the seeds start to pop. Mix in the turmeric and the chili powder; cook for fifteen seconds.

Mix in the potatoes, peas, salt, and jalapeño slices. (It is okay if the potatoes and the peas get a little smashed.) Turn off the heat, mix in the mint and lemon juice to taste, and save for later.

5. Roll the pastry until it is fairly thin (-inch thick). Cut roughly ten 6-inch circles from the dough. Cut each circle in half. Put a loaded tablespoon of filling in the middle of each half circle. Dampen the edges of the dough with cold water, fold the dough over on itself to make a triangle, and seal tightly.

6. To fry, put in roughly 3 inches of vegetable oil to a big deep cooking pan. Heat the oil using high heat until super hot, but not smoking. Put in the samosas to the hot oil a few at a time and deep-fry until a golden-brown colour is achieved. Using a slotted spoon, remove the samosas to a stack of paper towels to drain.

7. Serve the samosas with <u>Tamarind Dipping Sauce</u>.

Yield: 20 samosas

PUNJAB FISH

Ingredients:

- ¼ teaspoon cinnamon

- ¼ teaspoon saffron strands, toasted and crushed ½ cup
- plain yogurt

- 1 (1-inch) piece ginger, peeled and minced

- 1 clove garlic, chopped

- 1 medium onion, thinly cut

- 1 teaspoon black pepper

- 1 teaspoon salt

- 1 teaspoon turmeric

- 2 serrano chilies, seeded and minced

- 2 tablespoons almond slivers

- 2 tablespoons boiling water

- 2 teaspoons cardamom

- 2 teaspoons cumin

- 2–3 tablespoons vegetable oil

- 4–6 firm-fleshed fish fillets, roughly 1-inch thick Lemon juice

- teaspoon ground cloves

Directions:

1. Wash the fish with cold water and pat dry. Rub the fish with lemon juice.

2. Mix the salt, pepper, and turmeric; drizzle over the fish.

3. Heat one to 2 tablespoons of vegetable oil in a big frying pan using high heat. Brown the fish swiftly on each side. Take away the fish to a plate, cover, and save for later.

4. Put in the onion to the same pan and sauté until translucent and just starting to brown.

5. Put the cooked onion in a food processor together with the garlic, ginger, chilies, and almonds. Process to make a paste, putting in a small amount of water if required. Put in the cumin, cardamom, cinnamon, and clove; process to meticulously blend.

6. If required, put in additional vegetable oil to the frying pan to make about 2 tablespoons. Heat the oil over moderate. Put in the spice mixture and cook, stirring continuously, for approximately 2 minutes. Swirl a small amount of water in the food processor to remove any remaining spices and pour it into the pan; stir until blended.

7. Pour 2 tablespoons of boiling water into a small cup. Put in the toasted saffron and stir until blended. Pour the saffron water into the frying pan.

8. Mix in the yogurt. Heat to a simmer and allow the sauce to cook for five minutes.

9. Put in the fish to the sauce, flipping to coat. Cover and allow to simmer for roughly ten minutes or until the fish is done to your preference.

Yield: Servings 4–6

RED CURRY CAMBOGEE

Ingredients:

- 1 cup boiling water

- 2 tablespoons vegetable oil

- 4 cups Lemongrass Curry Sauce

- 4 dried Thai bird chilies, stemmed and seeded

- 4 tablespoons sweet paprika

Directions:

1. Break the dried chilies into pieces and put them in a small container. Cover with the boiling water and allow it to sit until soft, approximately fifteen minutes.

2. Put the chilies, their steeping water, and the paprika in a blender. Process to make a thin paste.

3. Heat the vegetable oil on moderate to high heat in a wok. Put in the chili paste and stir-fry until it starts to darken. Turn off the heat and save for later.

4. Put the Lemongrass Curry Sauce in a moderate-sized deep cooking pan. Mix in half of the chili paste and bring to its boiling point. Lower the heat and allow to simmer for five to ten minutes. Check the flavor of the sauce, putting in more chili paste if required.

Yield: Approximately 4½ cups

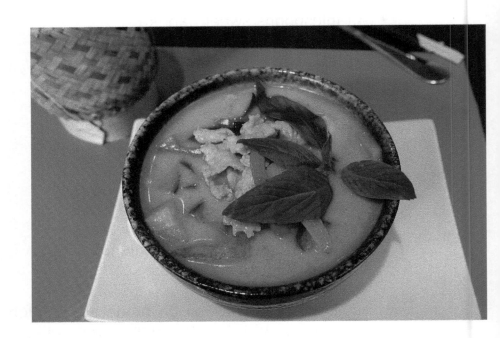

LEMONGRASS CURRY SAUCE

Ingredients:

- 1 cup chopped lemongrass, inner core only

- 1 teaspoon minced ginger

- 1 teaspoon turmeric

- 1 jalapeño chili, stemmed and seeded

- 3 small shallots, crudely chopped

- 3 (14-ounce) cans coconut milk

- 3 (2-inch-long, ½-inch wide) pieces lime peel
- ¼ teaspoon salt

- 4–5 cloves garlic, chopped

Directions:

1. Put the lemongrass, garlic, ginger, turmeric, chili, and shallots in a food processor; process to make a paste.

2. Bring the coconut milk to its boiling point and put in the lemongrass paste, lime peel,

and salt. Decrease the heat and allow to simmer for 30 to forty-five minutes. Take away the lime peel.

Yield: Approximately 4 cups

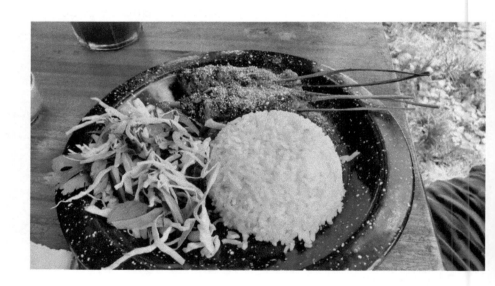

ROASTED DUCK, MELON, AND MANGO SALAD

Ingredients:

- ½ big cucumber, seeded and cut

- ½ roast duck, meat removed and shredded ½ teaspoon
- granulated salt ½
- teaspoon sesame oil

- 1 cup cubed cantaloupe

- 1 cup cubed honeydew melon

- 1 cup cubed jicama

- 1 mango, cut into bite-sized pieces

- 1 pear, cut into bite-sized pieces

- 1 tablespoon plus 2 teaspoons vegetable oil

- 1 teaspoon bottled chili sauce

- 1 teaspoon ketchup

- 1 teaspoon oyster sauce

- 1 teaspoon soy sauce

- 1 teaspoon sugar

- 1½ teaspoons apricot jam

- 1½ teaspoons cornstarch

- 2 tablespoons toasted sesame seeds

- 2 teaspoons fine sugar

- 3 tablespoons ground peanuts

- 3 tablespoons water

Directions:

1. In a moderate-sized-sized mixing container, mix the soy sauce, fine sugar, oyster sauce, and 1 tablespoon of the vegetable oil. Put in the shredded duck to the container and toss to coat; set aside.

2. In a small container, whisk together the 3 tablespoons of water, salt, 1 teaspoon of sugar, sesame oil, ketchup, chili sauce, and cornstarch; set aside.

3. In a small deep cooking pan, heat the rest of the vegetable oil on moderate heat. Put in the sauce mixture to the pan and cook until it becomes thick. Mix in the apricot jam and remove the pan from the heat. Cool the sauce in your fridge. Stir before you use.

4. Mound the duck in the middle of a big serving platter. Position the fruits and vegetables around the duck. Ladle the sauce over the duck, fruits, and vegetables. Drizzle the salad with chopped peanuts and sesame seeds. Serve immediately.

Yield: Servings 4–6

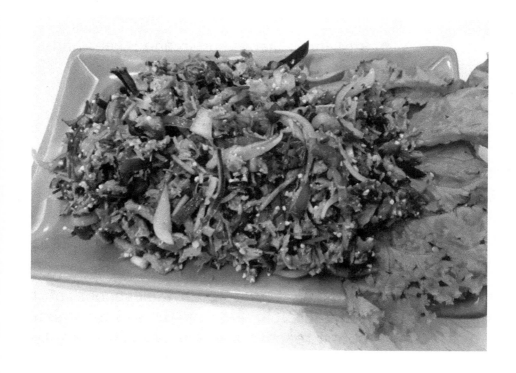

SHRIMP "PÂTÉ"

Ingredients:

- ¼ teaspoon white pepper

- ½ teaspoon salt

- 1 red chili, seeded and thoroughly minced (not necessary)

- 1 teaspoon sugar

- 1¼ cups minced shrimp

- 2 tablespoons vegetable oil

- 8 (4-inch) pieces sugarcane Sweet-and-sour or other favorite dipping sauce

Directions:

1. Preheat your oven to 375 degrees.

2. Put the shrimp, salt, sugar, white pepper, and chili in a food processor; process until the desired smoothness is achieved.

3. Sprinkle in one to 2 tablespoons of the vegetable oil. Process the shrimp mixture until it reaches the consistency necessary to make a meatball, using nearly oil.

4. Split the shrimp mixture into 4 equivalent portions.

5. Use your hands to mold a "shrimp ball" around the center of each of the sugarcane pieces.
6. Put the "skewers" on a baking sheet and roast for roughly twenty minutes. If you prefer them a little extra browned, broil them (after they are done baking) until the desired color is reached.

7. To serve, spoon some of the sweet-and-sour sauce into the middle of 4 plates. Put the sugarcane "skewer" on top of the sauce.

Yield: Servings 4

SINGAPORE NOODLES

Ingredients:

- ¼ cup oyster sauce

- 1 package rice sticks, soaked in hot water until tender and drained

- 1–2 teaspoons red pepper flakes

- 2 cups cooked meat or shrimp in bite-sized pieces

- 2 green onions, trimmed and thinly cut

- 2 tablespoons minced ginger

- 2 tablespoons vegetable oil

- 2 teaspoons soy sauce

- 3 tablespoons curry powder

- 4 cloves garlic, minced

Directions:

1. Heat the vegetable oil in a wok or big frying pan on moderate to high heat. Put in the garlic and the ginger. Stir-fry until tender.

2. Put in the cooked meat or shrimp, green onion, and red pepper flakes to the wok; stir-fry until hot.

3. Mix in the oyster sauce, curry powder, and soy sauce. Put in the rice noodles and toss. Serve instantly.

Yield: Servings 2–3

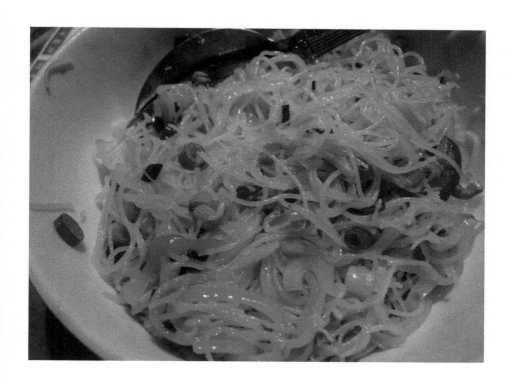

SINGAPORE SHELLFISH SOUP

Ingredients:

- ¼ cup chopped cilantro

- 1 (14-ounce) can coconut milk

- 1 (1-inch) piece ginger, peeled and chopped

- 1 7-ounce package of rice noodles, soaked in hot water until soft

- 1 cup bean sprouts

- 1 pound big raw shrimp, peeled, shells reserved

- 1 pound mussels, cleaned and debearded

- 1 tablespoon anchovy paste

- 1 tablespoon ground coriander

- 1 tablespoon lime zest

- 1 teaspoon turmeric

- 1–2 tablespoons fish sauce

- 2 cloves garlic, minced

- 2 tablespoons vegetable oil, divided

- 3 serrano chilies, seeded and chopped

- 3 stalks lemongrass, outer layers removed, inner core thinly cut

- 4 small shallots, peeled and cut

- 6 big scallops, cut horizontally into 2–3 pieces, depending on

  their size
- Lime wedges

Yield: Servings 6–8

Directions:

1. In a moderate-sized-sized deep cooking pan heat 1 tablespoon of the oil on moderate to high heat and fry the shrimp shells until pink.

2. Put in 3 cups of water to the pan and bring to its boiling point; decrease the heat and simmer for half an hour Strain the shells from the broth, then boil the broth until it is reduced to 2 cups.

3. In a big frying pan, bring ½ cup of water to its boiling point. Put in the mussels, cover, and allow to steam until opened,

approximately five minutes. Discard any mussels that have not opened. Strain the cooking liquid and save for later. Shell all but about of the mussels; set the mussels aside.

4. Put the lemongrass, chilies, garlic, ginger, shallots, anchovy paste, and 2 tablespoons of water in a food processor. Process to make a thick paste, putting in more water if required.

5. Heat the rest of the vegetable oil in a big soup pot on moderate heat. Put in the lemongrass paste and fry, stirring constantly, until mildly browned, approximately ten minutes. Mix in the turmeric and ground coriander and cook for a minute more.

6. Put in the shrimp broth and mussel cooking liquid to the pot, stirring to dissolve the paste. Bring to its boiling point, reduce heat, and simmer for ten to fifteen minutes.

7. Put in the coconut milk and fish sauce; return to its boiling point. Put in the noodles and lime zest; simmer for a couple of minutes. Put in the shrimp and simmer for a couple of minutes more. Put in the scallop slices. After half a minute or so, put in the shelled

mussels and bean sprouts. Lightly stir until blended.

8. To serve, ladle the soup into deep soup bowls. Decorate using the mussels in their shells, drizzle with chopped cilantro and the juice from a lime wedge over the top of each container.

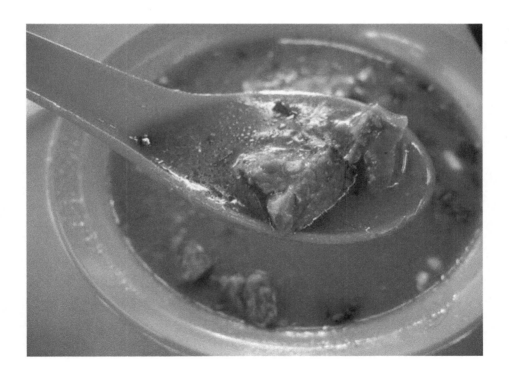

SINGAPORE SHRIMP

Ingredients:

- ¼ cup green onion slices

- ¼ teaspoon Chinese 5-spice powder

- 1 can coconut milk

- 1 clove garlic, minced

- 1 cup cut domestic mushrooms

- 1 teaspoon minced ginger

- 1½ pounds cooked shrimp

- 2 tablespoons vegetable oil

- 2 teaspoons hoisin sauce

- 2 teaspoons oyster sauce

- 2 teaspoons Red Curry Paste (Page 17)

- Salt and pepper to taste

Directions:

1. In a wok or big sauté pan, heat the vegetable oil on moderate to high.

2. Put in the mushrooms, green onions, garlic, and ginger; stir-fry for two to three minutes.

3. Mix together the hoisin sauce, oyster sauce, and curry paste, and 5-spice powder until well blended. Put in the mixture to the wok.

4. Mix in the coconut milk and tweak seasoning to taste with the salt and pepper. Put in the shrimp and bring to a simmer. Cook for one to two minutes until the shrimp are thoroughly heated.

Yield: Servings 4

SPICE-POACHED CHICKEN

Ingredients:

- ¼ cup light soy sauce

- ¼ teaspoon dried tangerine peel (dried orange peel can be substituted)

- ½ teaspoon whole black peppercorns

- ½ teaspoon whole cloves

- 1 (2-inch) cinnamon stick

- 1 cardamom pod

- 1 whole star anise

- 2 tablespoons sugar

- 4–6 boneless, skinless chicken breasts

- 5 cups water

Directions:

1. Put the star anise, peppercorns, cloves, cinnamon stick, cardamom pod, tangerine peel, and water in a stew pot. Bring the mixture to its boiling point using high heat. Let boil until the poaching liquid is reduced to 4 cups.

2. Mix in the soy sauce and the sugar. Return the liquid to its boiling point.

3. Put in the chicken breasts and reduce to a simmer. Poach the breasts until done, approximately twenty minutes.

Yield: Servings 4–6

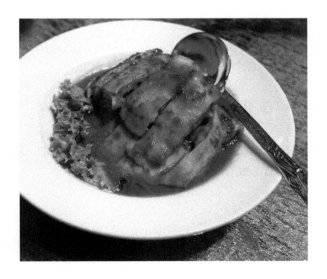

SWEET CAMBODIAN BROTH WITH PORK AND EGGS

Ingredients:

- ½ teaspoon freshly ground black pepper ½ teaspoon
- salt

- 1 big pork tenderloin, cut into bite-sized cubes

- 1 cup fish sauce

- 1 cup sugar

- 1 cup thinly cut bamboo shoots

- 4 cups water

- 5 tablespoons soy sauce

- 6–8 hard-boiled eggs

- Rice, cooked in accordance with package directions

Directions:

1. Bring the water to its boiling point in a big deep cooking pan. Put in the soy sauce, black pepper, salt, sugar, fish sauce, and hard-boiled eggs; simmer for fifteen minutes.

2. Put in the cubed pork and the bamboo shoots and simmer for another thirty minutes.

3. Lower the heat to low, cover, and allow to simmer for two to three hours. Adjust seasonings to taste.

4. To serve, mound some rice on the bottom of soup bowls. Ladle soup over the rice.

Yield: Servings 4–6

SWEET-AND-SOUR VEGETABLES

Ingredients:

- ¼ cup rice vinegar

- 1 big green pepper, seeded and slice into bite-sized pieces

- 1 cup brown sugar

- 1 cup cut carrots

- 1 cup fresh pineapple chunks

- 1 cup unsweetened pineapple juice

- 1 cup water, divided

- 1 onion, cut

- 1 teaspoon grated ginger

- 2 cloves garlic, crushed

- 2 tablespoons cornstarch

- 2 tablespoons soy sauce

- 4 cups broccoli

- 6 green onions, trimmed and slice into 1-inch lengths

Directions:

1. Put the carrots, onion, green pepper, garlic, and ginger in a big deep cooking pan with ½ cup of the water. Bring the water to its boiling point and allow to cook for five minutes, stirring regularly.

2. Put in the broccoli, green onions, and the rest of the ½ cup of water. Bring the water to its boiling point; reduce the heat, cover, and allow to simmer for five minutes.

3. In the meantime, in a small container, meticulously mix the pineapple juice, rice vinegar, soy sauce, brown sugar, and cornstarch.

4. Put in the pineapple juice mixture and the pineapple chunks to the wok. Raise the heat to moderate and cook, stirring continuously, until the sauce becomes thick.

Yield: Servings 6

TAMARIND DIPPING SAUCE

Ingredients:

- ½ teaspoon ground fennel

- 1 cup hot water

- 1 teaspoon ground cumin

- 1 teaspoon salt

- 2 teaspoons brown sugar

- 2 teaspoons grated ginger

- 3 tablespoons tamarind pulp

- Lemon juice to taste

Directions:

1. Put the tamarind pulp in a small container. Pour boiling water over the pulp and allow to soak until soft, approximately fifteen minutes.

2. Break up the pulp and then strain the tamarind water through a fine-mesh sieve,

using the back of a spoon to push the pulp through, but leaving the tough fibers.

3. Mix in the rest of the ingredients and let the tamarind sauce sit for minimum fifteen minutes before you serve.

Yield: Approximately 1¼ cups

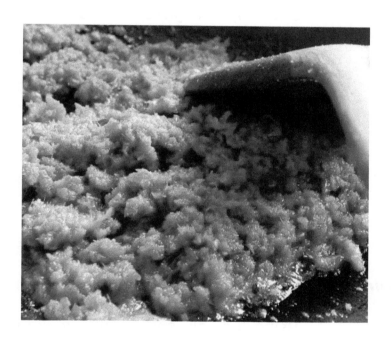

TANDOORI CHICKEN
Ingredients:

- ½ cup plain yogurt

- ½ teaspoon saffron threads

- 1 tablespoon grated ginger

- 1½ teaspoons <u>Garam Masala</u>

- 2 small garlic cloves, minced

- 2 tablespoons ghee, melted

- 2 teaspoons paprika

- 2 teaspoons salt

- 4 skinless chicken breasts

- 4 skinless chicken legs

- teaspoon chili powder

Directions:

1. Using a small, sharp knife, make three to 4 (¼-inch-deep) slits in each piece of chicken. Set aside in a container big enough to hold all of the pieces.

2. Put the saffron in a small sauté pan on moderate heat and toast for roughly half a minute. Put the saffron on a small plate and let it cool and crumble.

3. Mix the saffron into the yogurt.

4. Grind together the ginger, garlic, garlic, salt, chili pepper, paprika, and garam masala. Mix the spice mixture into the yogurt.

5. Pour the yogurt over the chicken, ensuring that all of the pieces are coated. Cover and marinate overnight flipping the pieces in the marinade every so frequently.

6. Preheat your oven to 450 degrees.

7. Put in the ghee to a roasting pan big enough to hold al of the chicken pieces. Put in the chicken, breast side down. Ladle some of the ghee over the pieces. Roast for about ten minutes. Turn the pieces over, coat again, and continue roasting for five minutes. Turn them again and roast for another five minutes. Turn 1 last time (breasts must be up); coat and cook until done, approximately 5 more minutes.

Yield: Servings 4

TEA-SMOKED CHICKEN

Ingredients:

- ½ cup brown sugar

- ½ cup cooked rice

- ½ cup green tea leaves

- ½ teaspoon salt

- 1 teaspoon sesame oil

- 2 teaspoons rice wine

- 6–8 boneless, skinless chicken breasts

Directions:

1. Swiftly wash the chicken breasts under cold water and pat dry. Drizzle with the salt and rice wine. Set aside in your fridge for half an hour

2. In the meantime, prepare the wok: Coat the bottom using a sheet of aluminium foil. Put the tea leaves, brown sugar, and rice on the bottom of the wok and toss to blend. Place a wire grill rack on the wok.

3. Heat the wok on moderate to high heat. Place the chicken on the rack and cover with a tight-fitting lid. Remove the heat after smoke starts to emit from the wok, but leave it on the burner for about ten minutes or until the chicken is thoroughly cooked.

4. Brush the chicken with the sesame oil. Serve immediately.

Yield: Servings 6–8

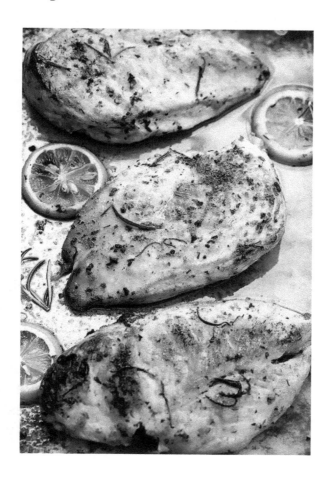

TROPICAL FRUITS WITH CINNAMON AND LIME

Ingredients:

- ½ teaspoon sesame oil

- ½–1 teaspoon cinnamon Pinch of salt

- 3 tablespoons honey

- 6 cups of tropical fruits, such as mango, papaya, bananas, melons, star fruit, kiwi, etc., (anything really) cut into bite-sized pieces

- Zest and juice of 6 limes

Directions:

1. Mix the lime zest and all but about of the lime juice in a small container. Slowly sprinkle in the honey, whisking to make a smooth mixture. Whisk in the sesame oil, cinnamon, and salt. Adjust flavor to your preference with more lime juice if required.

2. Put the fruit in a big serving container. Pour the cinnamon-lime dressing over the fruit, toss to blend, and allow to rest in your fridge for fifteen minutes before you serve.

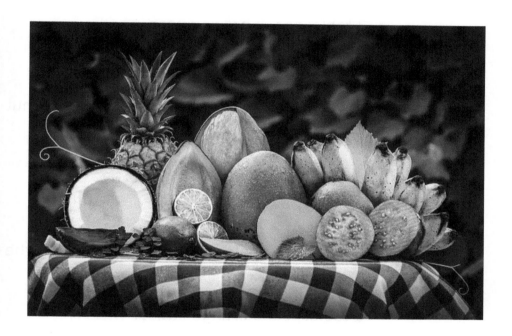

VIETNAMESE BANANAS

Ingredients:

- 1 tablespoon grated ginger Grated zest of 1 orange

- 3 tablespoons brown sugar

- 3 tablespoons butter

- 3 tablespoons shredded coconut (unsweetened)

- 3 teaspoons toasted sesame seeds

- 4 tablespoons lime juice

- 6 bananas, peeled and cut in half along the length

- 6 tablespoons orange liqueur

Directions:

1. Heat a small nonstick pan using high heat. Put in the coconut and cook, stirring continuously, until a golden-brown colour is achieved. Take away the coconut from the pan and save for later.

2. In a big sauté pan, melt the butter on moderate to high heat. Mix in the brown sugar, the ginger, and orange zest. Put the bananas in the pan, cut-side down, and cook for one to two minutes or until the sauce begins to become sticky. Turn the bananas over to coat in the sauce. Put the bananas on a heated serving platter and cover using aluminium foil.

3. Return the pan to the heat and meticulously mix in the lime juice and the orange liqueur. Using a long-handled match, ignite the sauce. Allow the flames to die down and then pour the sauce over the bananas.

4. Drizzle the bananas with the toasted coconut and the sesame seeds. Serve instantly.

Yield: Servings 6

VIETNAMESE OXTAIL SOUP

Ingredients:

- ¼ cup chopped cilantro

- ½ pound bean sprouts

- 1 (7-ounce) package rice sticks, soaked in hot water until tender and drained

- 1 green onion, trimmed and thinly cut

- 1 small cinnamon stick

- 1 tablespoon vegetable oil

- 1 tablespoon whole black peppercorns

- 1 whole star anise

- 2 garlic cloves, peeled and crushed

- 2 limes, cut into wedges

- 2 medium carrots, peeled and julienned

- 2 medium onions

- 3 tablespoons fish sauce

- 4 (½-inch) pieces ginger, peeled

- 4 serrano chilies, seeded and thinly cut

- 5 pounds meaty oxtails

- Freshly ground black pepper to taste

Directions:

1. Cut 1 of the onions into ¼-inch slices. Heat the vegetable oil in a moderate-sized sauté pan on moderate to high heat. Put in the onion slices and sauté until they barely start to brown. Drain the oil from the browned onion and save for later.

2. Slice the rest of the onion into paper-thin slices. Cover using plastic wrap and save for later.

3. Wash the oxtails in cold water and put them in a stock pot. Cover the tails with cold water and bring to its boiling point. Lower the heat and skim any residue that has come to the surface. Let simmer for fifteen minutes.

4. Put in the browned onions, ginger, carrots, cinnamon, star anise, peppercorns, and garlic. Return the stock to a simmer and cook for 6 to 8 hours, putting in water if required.

5. When the broth is done, skim off any additional residue. Take away the oxtails from the pot and allow to cool until easy to handle. Take away the meat from the bones. Position the meat on a platter and decorate it with the cut green onions. Discard the bones.

6. Strain the broth and return to the stove. Put in the fish sauce and black pepper to taste. Keep warm.

7. On a second platter, position the bean sprouts, chopped cilantro, cut chilies, and lime wedges.

8. Bring a pot of water to its boiling point. Plunge the softened rice noodles in the water to heat. Drain.

9. To serve, place a portion of the noodles in each container. Set a tureen of the broth on the table together with the platter of oxtail meat and the platter of accompaniments. Let your guests serve themselves.

Yield: Servings 6–8

VIETNAMESE PORK STICKS

Ingredients:

For the pork:

- ¼ teaspoon Chinese hot chili oil

- ¼ teaspoon sugar

- ½ cup chopped basil

- ½ cup chopped cilantro

- ½ cup chopped mint

- 1 (½-inch) piece ginger, peeled and minced

- 1 clove garlic, minced

- 1 green onion, trimmed and minced

- 1 pound lean ground pork

- 1 tablespoon soy sauce

- 1¼ teaspoons lemon juice

- 12 bamboo skewers, soaked in water

    12 Boston or leaf lettuce leaves

-

- 2 teaspoons vegetable oil

- 6 big water chestnuts, minced

- teaspoon salt

For the dipping sauce:

- ½ cup soy sauce

- 1 (1-inch) piece ginger, minced

- 1 teaspoon oyster sauce

- 2 garlic cloves, minced

- 2 teaspoons sugar

- 3 tablespoons water

- 5 tablespoons lemon juice

- Pinch of cayenne pepper

Directions:

1. To prepare the pork: In a big container, use your hands to meticulously mix the ground pork, water chestnuts, garlic, green onion,

soy sauce, vegetable oil, lemon juice, ginger, sugar, chili oil, and salt.

2. Split the mixture into 12 portions. Shape each portion into a cylinder about 3 inches by 1 inch. Cautiously insert a bamboo skewer through each cylinder along the length. Set aside.

3. Put the lettuce leaves, cilantro, mint, and basil in 4 separate serving bowls. Place in your fridge until ready to serve.

4. To prepare the dipping sauce: In a small deep cooking pan mix all the sauce ingredients. Bring the mixture to its boiling point on moderate to high heat. Decrease the heat and simmer for five minutes. Take away the sauce from the heat and allow to cool.

5. Prepare a charcoal or gas grill. Put the skewers in a grill basket, ensuring they are tightly held but not squashed. Grill the skewers until the pork is thoroughly cooked and the outside is crunchy, approximately ten to fifteen minutes flipping the basket regularly.

6. To serve, pour each guest some of the dipping sauce into a small individual container. Put the bowls of cilantro, mint, and basil in the center of the table. Put 2

lettuce leaves and 2 pork skewers on each guest's plate.

7. To assemble, have each guest slide the pork from the skewer onto a lettuce leaf. Drizzle the pork with some of the herbs to taste. Roll the lettuce around the pork and dip in the sauce.

Yield: Servings

Lightning Source UK Ltd.
Milton Keynes UK
UKHW020651300421
382894UK00005B/61